Alzheimer's or Dementia

What to do
when your loved one is diagnosed

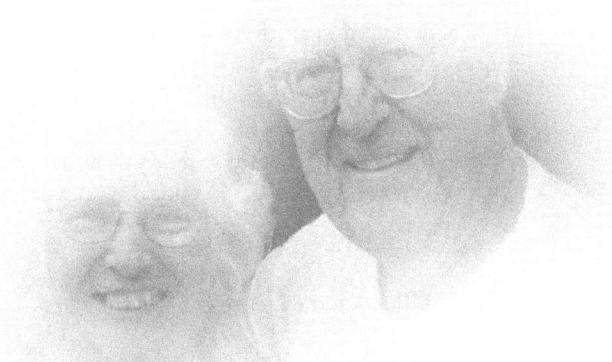

MARK HIEBERT

ISBN 13: 978-1500798857

Printed in the United States of America

First Printing: 2015

19 18 17 16 15   5 4 3 2 1

Cover and interior design by James Monroe Design, LLC.

133 Martesia Way
Indian Harbour Beach, FL 32937

For more information please visit:
www.AlzheimersOrDementia.org

To order visit: Amazon.com

*This book is dedicated to my wife Linda
who works very hard to keep her parents
safe and happy.*

Acknowledgments

My sincerest gratitude goes out to Janet Steiner, Jan McCarter, Aprille Waltrop, Tracy Budesa, and Debbie Shepherd for their help in contributing comments and reviewing the manuscript for this book. Their efforts made this book much more accurate and relevant for those with loved ones that have recently been diagnosed with Alzheimer's and other types of Dementia.

Welcome

As this guide goes to print many changes are occur-
ring within our health care system; it was written with
this in mind. The steps and agency contacts are presented in a way to be applicable even after changes
are made. The Patient Protection and Affordable Care
Act of 2010 or "Obamacare" is starting to have an
impact to the health care industry. As with any health
care program, changes will continue to take place.
We have tried to reflect the latest known changes, but
the Patient Protection and Affordable Care Act will
continue to impact the health care system for years to
come.

Contents

Introduction

Welcome to the How-To guide for caregivers when your loved one is diagnosed with Alzheimer's or other forms of Dementia. This guide is not designed to address each and every question you may encounter, rather it is meant to provide you with a big-picture roadmap that will take you through the maze of programs, Health Maintenance Organizations and Preferred Provider Organizations and agencies that can provide the different kinds of aid that are out there for you and your family members; see terms HMOs/PPOs (healthcare corporations that are financed by paying healthcare insurance premiums). This guide is provided as a checklist to assist in your effort to obtain the aid that will help you cope with the sometimes difficult task of caring for your loved one as well as YOURSELF. It is written in general terms so you can easily follow the steps through the maze of agencies you will encounter in your search to find the best and most affordable care for your loved one. Please read through this guide before accomplishing any steps. Some of the steps can be accomplished simultaneously, and others need to be followed in sequence. After you read through this guide and understand the process, hopefully you will have a better understanding of the steps as they are presented.

The agencies you need to work with may be different depending on which healthcare provider you choose and which state and county your family member lives in, but we have gone to great effort to include information on those agencies that we found the most helpful in Florida. **Although this guide is primarily written for residents of Florida, the principles/steps are universal, no matter where your family member lives.** Examples of aid available to qualified individuals include, but are not limited to: Care or Case Management, Home Health Care, Adult Day Care, Chore Services, Home Delivered Meals, Caregiver Respite, Home Companion Care, Hearing, Vision and Dental Screening, Assisted Living Facilities, and Nursing Facility Services.

This can be an extremely difficult time for you and your loved one. Your journey will be a lot smoother if you have a helpful and reliable partner, friend or other family member to assist you. There is a light at the end of the tunnel, and hopefully this guide will save you countless hours of frustration on your journey to get the best care for your loved one.

Note: The information presented in this guide is for the layperson and is a result of actual experience. The author is not a legal or medical expert and as such the reader is reminded to consult a qualified legal and/ or medical advisor for their particular expertise.

The steps listed below will be discussed in further detail.

Step 1 - Identify and make an appointment with your loved one's Healthcare provider

Step 2 - Determine your loved ones eligibility for enrollment in MEDICARE

Step 3 - Make an appointment with a lawyer familiar in Elder Law

Step 4 - Get a complete geriatric health evaluation

Step 5 - Contact the Florida Department of Elder Affairs or your State's Area Agency on Aging to see what programs your loved one may be qualified for

Step 6 - Determine living/housing arrangements—your needs

Step 7 - Match your financial ability with your needs

Step 8 - Investigate other Aid Programs

Identify and make an appointment with
your loved one's Healthcare provider

Determine your loved ones eligibility
for enrollment in MEDICARE

Make an appointment with
a lawyer familiar in Elder Law

Get a complete geriatric
health evaluation

Contact your State's
Area Agency on Aging
to see available programs

Determine living/housing
arrangements-your needs

Match your financial
ability with your needs

Investigate other
Aid Programs

Step 1

Identify and make an appointment with your loved one's Healthcare provider.

Chances are your loved one has already been diagnosed with a memory impaired condition or you would not be reading this guide. Who is your loved one's primary care physician (PCP)? Hopefully your loved one's doctor has already referred them to a specialist who is a brain health expert, or a Geriatric provider who specializes in dementia-related illnesses. If your loved one does not yet have a PCP, choosing one that is knowledgeable in treating elderly patients would be very helpful to both you and your loved one.

Step 2

Determine your loved one's eligibility for enrollment in MEDICARE.

If he/she is eligible for MEDICARE, (age 65 or older), make sure you assist them in applying for MEDICARE. Your loved one can apply for MEDICARE three months prior to their 65th birthday by going to the Social Security website at www.socialsecurity.gov, by phone at 1-800-772-1213, or you can visit your local Social Security Administration office. The website or telephone contact is generally faster and easier than visiting in person. More information on MEDICARE is listed under Social Security and MEDICARE (Step 8). Note that MEDICARE annually offers open enrollment from mid-October through December, at which time your loved one can change providers for any reason. Always check with your MEDICARE Office or website for enrollment times or changes.

What are your MEDICARE coverage choices?

There are two main choices of MEDICARE coverage. The steps below will help with this decision.

Decide if you want Original MEDICARE or a MEDICARE Advantage Plan

Original Medicare

- Includes Part A (Hospital insurance) and/or Part B (Medical insurance)
- MEDICARE provides this coverage directly.
- Choices of doctors, hospitals, and other providers that accept MEDICARE.
- You or your supplemental coverage pay deductibles and coinsurance.
- You usually pay a monthly premium for Part B (Medical insurance).

Decide if you need prescription drug coverage (Part D)

If you want drug coverage you must join a MEDI-CARE Prescription Drug Plan, and you will usually pay a monthly premium. These plans are run by private companies approved by MEDICARE.

If you choose Original MEDICARE, decide whether you want a Supplemental Coverage

- You may want to get coverage that fills gaps in Original MEDICARE coverage. You can choose to buy a MEDICARE Supplemental Insurance (MEDIGAP) policy from a private company. Costs vary by policy and company.

- You may find Employers/Unions may offer similar coverage.

MEDICARE Supplement insurance policies (sometimes called MEDIGAP) are sold by private insurance companies, and help pay some of the costs MEDICARE may not cover. There are sign-up time restrictions such as a one-time six-month MEDIGAP "open enrollment" period which starts the first month you are 65; check the MEDICARE website or call for more information or for any changes.

MEDICARE Advantage Plan (HMO/PPO) / Part C includes BOTH Part A and Part B.

- Private insurance companies approved by MEDICARE provide this coverage.

- Generally you need to use plan doctors, hospitals, and other providers, or you may pay more or all of the costs.

- You might pay a monthly premium (in addition to your Part B premium) and a copayment or coinsurance for covered services; varies by state.

- Costs, extra coverage and rules vary by plan and state.

Decide if you need prescription drug coverage (Part D)

- If you want prescription drug coverage and it's offered by your plan, in most cases you must get it through your plan.
- In some types of plans that don't offer drug coverage, you can join a MEDICARE Prescription Drug Plan.

This is a brief summary of the two main MEDI-CARE options, but it is not comprehensive. There are many more issues and decisions to be made regarding your MEDICARE and Supplemental Insurance options and other MEDICARE options. Contact your local social security office or visit www.medicare.gov to get more in-depth information.

For more information, contact your State Health Insurance Assistance Program (SHIP). SHIPs are state programs that get money from the federal government to give local health insurance counseling to people with MEDICARE. **SHIPs are not connected to any insurance company or health plan. SHIP volunteers work hard to help you with the following MEDICARE questions or concerns:**

- Plan choices
- How MEDICARE works with other insurance
- Your MEDICARE rights
- Billing problems
- Complaints about your medical care or treatment

In Florida, your SHIP is the Department of Elder Affairs. One of the programs the Department of Elder Care administers is Serving Health Insurance Needs of Elders (**SHINE**). **This program can provide you with free counseling and information on MEDICARE supplemental plans. They do not sell anything, but they can help you navigate the different MEDI-CARE plan options and other programs. You can contact them at www.floridashine.org or 1-800-963-5337. They may have to call you back but their help is second to none. They are there to help you and your family member. SHINE services are free, unbiased and confidential.**

Step 3

Make an appointment with a Lawyer familiar in elder care law.

If you have not yet done so, you will need to discuss with your loved one who he/she wants designated to act as their trusted agent for legal, financial, and medical decisions. This should be either a trusted family member or friend; your family member will need to designate this person as legal representative by getting a legal *Durable Power of Attorney*. This will give the legal representative the right to make decisions for your family member that, with the further progression of their dementia, he/she may not be able to make competently. Your loved one can designate more than one person to have *Durable Power of Attorney*, due to distance between family members and/or a delegation of certain functions among several people. For example, one person could make medical decisions and another, financial decisions.

Make an appointment with a law firm that is familiar with elder law. The lawyer can assist you in itemizing your family member's assets and income. They may also help to determine any asset redistribution options available to your family member. There are a lot of misunderstandings regarding this legal step, and there are very strict laws dealing with assets that can and cannot be "redistributed." A lawyer will advise you on the legal guidelines when discussing your family member's financial options. These legal policies can vary from state to state and even between counties. Don't be intimidated by the fear of paying inflated lawyer fees; this step could very well be a great investment by saving you money as you attempt to navigate this legal jungle. There are also free legal services that you can contact. Florida Senior Legal agencies are: Brevard County Legal Aid at www.brevardcountylegalaid.org or 321-631-2500, or Florida Senior Legal Helpline at 1-888-895-7873. You can reach the Florida Bar Lawyer Referral Service at www.flabar.org or 1-800-342-8011 (will charge a $25 fee for a 30 minute consultation). There are also websites that offer some of these legal documents for the do-it-yourselfer. More information and sample documents are available from the website: www.ahca.myflorida.com. Select publications from the pull down menu and search for Health Care Advance Directives.

Documents the Primary Caregiver should have:

Specific documents at a minimum the lawyer should recommend (other documents may be needed depending on your family member's assets, estate, etc.): *Living Will, Last Will and Testament, Durable Power of Attorney* and *Designation of Healthcare Surrogate.*

Living Will - Specifies what actions should be taken for your family member's health if he/she is no longer able to make decisions due to illness or incapacity. This document appoints someone to make such decisions on his/her behalf.

Last Will and Testament - Specifies the last wishes of the family member in regard to their possessions. It designates a person to manage the estate and provides for the transfer of the property at death.

Durable Power of Attorney Contingent upon Incapacity - Appoints a person to represent or act on another's behalf in private affairs, business, or other legal matters.

Designation of Healthcare Surrogate - Designates a surrogate for health care decisions in the event your family member has been determined to be incapacitated, in order to provide informed consent for medical treatment and surgical and diagnostic procedures.

Other documents: Do Not Resuscitate order (DNR) if desired - this document must be completed by your family member's Primary Care Physician.

Step 4

Get a complete Geriatric Health Evaluation.

If your family member has never had a "geriatric" evaluation, make an appointment with a Geriatric Specialist **for a complete Geriatric health evaluation**. This step can be crucial to the Caregiver and family member. Your family member's Primary Care Provider may be able to provide a referral to a specialist, although you do not need a referral to make an appointment. In Brevard County, Florida, some of the better known geriatric centers are the Health First Aging Institute *at 321-453-7100,* Parrish Senior Solutions at 321-268-6800, or your area's Aging Services. If your family member does not yet have a medical Diagnosis of Condition from the family doctor (Alzheimer's or other form of dementia), a geriatric specialist can make this diagnosis through an extremely thorough examination process. **This is an important step, as you will need a doctor's medical diagnosis when requesting aid for your family member based on a diagnosis of alzheimer's/dementia.**

Note: **Ensure that your family member's PCP and the Geriatric Specialist accept your family member's medical coverage (i.e. private insurance, MEDICARE, and/or MEDICARE supplement plan).** If your family member has an insurance that the geriatric specialist does not accept, he/she can self-pay; this can be expensive, depending on what treatment your family member may need. You may submit the bill to your private insurance company to see if they will pay all or a portion of the bill, but **check with your insurance in advance.** The Geriatric Specialist may recommend referrals for further diagnostic tests or treatment based on the exam (i.e., brain MRI or other brain scan, Physical Therapy, Speech Therapy, etc.). Each healthcare network (HMO, PPO or other organization) has its own network of doctors and specialists. **If you become aware of a particular doctor you want to see, make sure he/she accepts your health insurance.** These doctors will become part of your family member's medical team. **With their help, you and your family member can determine their healthcare needs and to what degree you may need help in meeting those needs. In Florida, if you are looking for financial aid with the cost of an Assisted Living Facility (ALF), an Agency for**

Health Care Administration (AHCA) Form 1823 will need to be completed by your family member's physician prior to or within 30 days of admission to an assisted living facility.

Step 5

Contact the Aging and Disability Resource Center (ADRC) or your State's Area Agency on Aging to see what programs your loved one may qualify for.

Don't wait for the Geriatric health evaluation process to slow you down, call this agency as soon as possible to get the ball rolling. Once you initially contact ADRC you will ask for assistance either in the home or with an ALF, based on your loved one's needs (Step 4). If you cannot get a referral operator on the phone, leave a message. They should contact you in the next 7 to 10 days and will conduct a telephone assessment, known as Department of Elder Affairs (DOEA) Form 701A. You should have your loved one's general financial information available at this time, as their total monthly income has to be below a given amount as designated by the State before they can qualify for financial assistance or services from the State. Some of the financial information the ADRC will require for this initial assessment: any social security payments, VA benefits (if applicable), bank account statements with total amounts, any investment accounts, retirement benefits, and any other assets or property, such as a home. You will also need to have the individual joint income levels. If you need help in compiling these documents, refer to a lawyer familiar with elder law (Step 3) or an agency in the community; the ADRC may be able to recommend someone to help. However, a lawyer familiar with elder care law is highly recommended.

After the initial phone assessment, a comprehensive medical assessment or Level of Care (LOC) assessment (Florida MEDICAID Form 3008) will be completed to assess your loved one's health, environment, social resources, mental status, nutrition and caregiver needs. If your loved one initially qualifies for one of the State programs, ADRC will refer your contact information to the Department of Elder Affairs and your family member will be assigned a caseworker who will set up an appointment to interview you (as the primary caregiver) and your family member to determine their care giving needs, known as DOEA Form 701B (usually accomplished where your family member resides). The caseworker will present several brochures for independent organizations/programs within your county that are contracted with the DOEA. The Department of Elder Affairs caseworker can assess for long term senior care, and coordinate primary care. This two part assessment process can take up to 6 months or longer, so patience and perseverance are important in the effort to gain assistance for your loved one. After the assessment is completed and the ADRC has the information it needs confirming your loved one qualifies for State assistance (DOEA Forms 701A, 701B and Florida MEDICAID Form 3008) your loved one is placed on a wait list for the program that you and your loved one have chosen. If your loved ones additionally qualify for MEDICAID coverage, the ADRC will mail a MEDICAID Access Application to apply for MEDICAID (this will be mailed to you as their caregiver, so make sure they have a correct address)— **it is important to fill this out completely.** Once the ADRC has received the application and documents you provide, you may be contacted several times with requests to provide additional documentation or information that they need to complete their review of the application. If and when your loved ones MEDICAID application has been approved, MEDICAID will backdate the coverage to the date that they initially received the application. The goal of the Long Term Senior Care Program is to keep your family member(s) in their home (or an Assisted Living Facility or the least restrictive environment), when appropriate. It also stretches the dollars allocated for these state programs, as a nursing home is a much more expensive alternative to assistance in the home or an ALF.

The process, forms and types of assessments can change, so be sure to ask your caseworker and the agency you are working what is the next step; keep in touch with them, as these forms have been known to get stuck or can be initially denied even though the requirements for state assistance have been met. This is the most challenging part of this process. **Note**: This step took the author's family over 6 months with repeated requests for additional or more in-depth information from the state agency before our loved ones were finally approved for financial assistance and healthcare aid from the state. SO KEEP TRYING AND DON'T GIVE UP!!

Step 6

*Determining Living/Housing
Arrangements-your needs*

Is your family member able to live on their own with part-time caregiver support or possibly a full-time, live in caregiver? Or would an Assisted Living Facility be the better choice? Does your family member need 24/7 nursing support such as provided by a permanent Nursing Facility?

If you decide on either an Assisted Living Facility or a Nursing home, ensure that you check the State's oversight or "watchdog" agency. In Florida this oversight agency is the Florida Agency for Health Care Administration (AHCA). This agency will give you information about how the facility is run, a 'report card' on how well the residents/patients are treated. Also, visit several facilities before making a decision; talk with the residents, visit at different times. There is also a program called Ombudsman, made up of trained volunteers that protect and ensure patient's rights by addressing patient concerns in nursing homes, assisted living facilities, and adult family care facilities. All services are confidential and free of charge. If you are asking for financial aid with an ALF, your program caseworker will give you a list of facilities that their program has contracted with. Depending on the facility and your family member's care needs, room and board could range from $2500 to $6000+ a month. A complete list of ALFs and Nursing Homes can be found online at www.floridahealthfinder.gov.

Keep in mind that your loved one's medical and care giving requirements will increase as dementia progresses, thus his/her needs should be reviewed regularly by their doctor and the staff at the facility you choose; also, as care giving needs increase, so may the monthly cost of the assistance given at the ALF. When looking for a facility, typically the monthly charge for the room consists of a flat room fee and a fee assessed by the number of services needed. The level of care required by each resident will be determined through a personal assessment done by the ALF staff. They will design a plan to provide customized services and quality care suited for each resident. Rates are based on accommodations and required services to satisfy the needs of each resident. The level of care is determined by a list of Activities of Daily Living (ADLs), a term in healthcare that refers to daily self-care activities within an individual's place of residence. Basic ADLs consist of self-care tasks such as: personal hygiene and grooming, dressing and undressing, self-feeding, functional transfers (getting into and out of bed or wheelchair, getting onto or off toilet, etc.), bowel and bladder management, and ambulation (walking with or without use of an assistive device such as a walker, cane or crutches; need for assistance with a wheel-chair). As the resident's care giving needs increase, so, too, may the fees. You need to ensure that when you are negotiating a contract with a facility that all the associated costs are spelled out, and that you under-stand when there might be an increase in the monthly fee due to an increase in the level of care needs.

Note: The financial determination will be based on your family member's financial situation including income and assets. The caregiver's finan-cial situation is not part of the assessment, unless the caregiver is the spouse of the family member, then the financial situation is based on joint incomes. The more income or financial assets your family member has, the less **FINANCIAL** aid they may qualify for. **Check with your lawyer/legal represen-tative for this determination (Step 3).** However, the Ombudsman program also has an array of services it will provide based on your family member's individual needs. The program can assist you and your family member in coping with the many aspects of care giving and home health care. Examples of services available to you and your family member may include: Care or Case Management, Home Health Care, Adult Day Care, Chore Services, Consumable Medical Supplies,

Home Delivered Meals, Emergency Response System, Family/Caregiver Training Services, Transportation to Medical Appointments, Caregiver Respite, Hearing, Vision and Dental Screening, Assisted Living Facility services, Nursing Facility Services and more.

If you have not made an appointment with an Elder Law Lawyer (Step 3), do it now. This is money well spent and will assist you in determining your options.

Step 7.

Match your financial ability with your needs.

Once you have a medical diagnosis, a list of state and county aid available, your needs identified in providing assistance, and your legal paperwork, you should take the time to sit down and make sure you are clear on the process so far. This stressful process will be made simpler if you understand where you are, how you got there, and where to go from here. You now should have all the pieces to proceed with deciding what options are best for you and your family member.

At this point, you need to determine your loved one's income level. Take the monthly amount of financial aid the state or county will provide and add your family member's gross monthly income. Please note, the difference between the main income level and your needs is not the end of the story. Now, let's look at the many different independent aid programs to try to make up some of the difference between the main income and your monthly financial needs (the costs of your family member's needs).

Step 8.

Investigate other Aid Programs.

This step lists some of the different aid programs you can contact to see if your family member qualifies for financial aid or other assistance.

Social Security Administration

The Social Security Administration is the government agency that administers some of the different state programs such as MEDICARE and MEDICAID.

MEDICARE Application

If your family member is close to 65 but not getting Social Security benefits, and he/she wants Part A and Part B, he/she will need to sign up. Call Social Security at 1-800-772-1213 or visit your local Social

Security Office for more information about MEDI-CARE eligibility and to sign up for Part A and Part B. You can also get general information about enrolling at www.medicare.gov. Personalized health care counseling at no cost from your State Health Insurance Assistance Program is also available. In Florida, call Serving Health Insurance Needs of Elders (SHINE) at 1-800-963-5337, or at www.floridashine.org/.

MEDICARE

MEDICARE is a national health insurance program for anyone 65 years or older (or people under 65 with certain disabilities) that contains four parts, A through D. It is a program the Social Security Administration administers. Original MEDICARE, sometimes called "fee-for-service" MEDICARE, includes Parts A and B (below).

Part A is a hospital insurance program that helps cover inpatient care in hospitals, skilled nursing facility care, hospice care, and home health care.

Part B is a medical insurance program that helps cover services from doctors and other health care providers, outpatient care, home health care, durable medical equipment, and some preventative services.

Part C is a MEDICARE Advantage option that is run by MEDICARE-approved private insurance companies, including all benefits and services covered under Parts A and B. It usually includes MEDICARE prescription drug coverage (Part D) as part of the plan, and may include extra benefits and services for an additional cost. Part C is like an HMO (Health Maintenance Organization) or PPO (Preferred Provider Organization). Part C combines Part A, Part B and usually Part D.

Part D is a prescription drug program that is run by MEDICARE-approved private insurance companies, and helps cover the cost of prescription drugs. It may help lower prescription drug costs and help protect against higher costs in the future.

MEDICAID

MEDICAID is a joint federal and state program that helps pay medical costs if you have limited income and resources and meet other state requirements. Medicaid programs differ from state to state, and each state has different income and resource requirements. Some people qualify for both MEDICARE and MEDICAID and are called "dual eligible." MEDICAID can be a supplement to MEDICARE. If your family member has MEDICARE and full MEDICAID coverage, most of their health care costs are covered. Also with MEDICARE and full MEDICAID, MEDICARE covers the Part D prescription drugs. Persons with MEDICAID may get some types of coverage that MEDICARE may not cover such as nursing home care and personal care services. Contact your state Aging and Disability Resource Center (ADRC) through your state Senior Resource Alliance (SRA) to get information about available programs in your area at www.seniorresourcealliance.org or 1-800-963-5337.

Florida Department of Elder Affairs (Serving Healthcare Insurance Needs of Elders - SHINE) is **your one-stop shop for in-depth, free and accurate advice on MEDICARE, MEDICAID and MEDICARE Supplement Health Insurance**. Their free advice by trained volunteers is available and open to all. Contact them at 1-800-963-5337 or at www.floridashine.org.

Veterans Affairs (VA)

If your family member is a Veteran, has ever served in the US Military, or is retired military, contact your local VA facility. **Generally, your family member's condition would have to be service-related (caused by military service) to qualify for benefits, unless they are retired from active duty.**

See your VA Primary Care Physician (VA PCP) and bring your family member's medical history and DD Form 214 (a Government form that proves service in military). If you don't have a DD-214, apply with the VA to get a copy.

VA aid could range from a monthly stipend or hearing aids to Respite where the VA will give you a small respite (up to 2 weeks) depending on what the family member (vet) qualifies for. Factors that impact what aid the family member may qualify for include income level, dates of service, service related injuries, etc.

In certain circumstances, spouses could qualify for aid under the Aid and Attendance program. Again, contact the VA for more information as many factors come into play for this program.

Note: The VA offers good programs, but the wheels of government programs turn slowly. If you do engage the VA, the normal turn-around time is usually months rather than days or weeks. Engage early and have patience. There are good programs if you qualify! Visit www.va.gov or call 1-800-827-1000.

Federal Employee Health Benefits Program (FEHB)

FEHB Health coverage is for current and retired federal employees and covered family members. They usually have their own prescription° drug program so the family member doesn't need to join a MEDICARE drug plan.

Visit www.opm/insure or call 1-800-878-5707.

Department of Defense (TRICARE for Life)

If your family member has been in the US Military, you can get TRICARE (free if on Active Duty). Military retirees and their families can qualify for TRICARE for Life health care program. Most people with TRICARE who are entitled to Part A must have Part B (MEDICARE) to keep TRICARE prescription drug benefits. To reach TRICARE visit www.tricare4u.com or call 1-866-773-0404.

OUR STORY

My wife, Linda, recently moved her parents, Gene and Bernice, to Florida from Washington State. Both had been diagnosed with Memory-Impaired conditions (Bernice with Alzheimer's and Gene with Dementia) by their family doctor in Washington. Gene and Bernice were starting to lose their abilities to function on their own without assistance, so their seven children got together and discussed their current living and financial circumstances with them, and they made the decision to move to Florida to be closer to Linda, who was chosen to be their Primary Caregiver. They arrived in Florida in May of 2012, and Linda and I went to work. Linda took over her parents' finances and made an appointment with an Elder Care Lawyer. We found an Alzheimer's Caregiver's support group at our local church, and we started to attend the monthly meetings. These meetings were invaluable to us in the beginning, as they provided great advice on where to start for aid and assistance; the group is made up of wonderful and warm people who had first-hand experience as the primary caregivers for their spouses and family members, and it was a relief to share our frustrations and issues with a group that had been there and gone through what we were currently experiencing. However, we found that there were no real guidelines of what to do, when to do it, or why; just information that wasn't organized into any type of a guideline or "to do" list. We attended different support group meetings but the lack of a caregiver's guide made life and the way to proceed at that time very frustrating and worrisome.

Linda spent many days on the phone with different agencies, not knowing where she was in the process, and which direction to go. Thankfully, her employer was very generous and supportive and granted her the time to pursue this endeavor. She researched her parents' current health program and confirmed they were enrolled in a MEDICARE Advantage plan in Washington. She transferred their MEDICARE Advantage program to Florida. Remember, the MEDICARE Advantage premiums and programs vary from State to State, and your family member must have coverage depending on what state/region they live in. She spoke with their MEDICARE Advantage insurance company that insured them in Washington, and changed their program to cover them in Florida. **Steps 1 and 2 were done**.

Having identified her parents' Healthcare Insurance provider, Linda then needed to find a new PCP for her parents, one that was familiar in elder care medicine and also accepted their insurance. After that, she enrolled her parents in an Adult Day Care program, and the staff there informed her of a geriatric doctor that worked in conjunction with the family PCP to provide an in-depth geriatric evaluation and provide a more complete diagnosis of condition. Linda called the Health First Institute for Aging and made appointments for both her parents (there is a substantial waiting period for this provider, the first appointment available for them was 3 months); she provided medical records from their previous doctor in Washington with the diagnosis for both Gene and Bernice. After the initial examination process, the Geriatric Specialist confirmed Bernice's diagnosis of Alzheimer's, and Gene's diagnosis was further classified as Frontal Temporal Dementia (a year later the diagnosis was further defined as Alzheimer's with a frontal temporal dimension). The doctor then referred them to various specialists and therapists that would assist in getting a more complete picture of where the parents were in the progression of their diseases, and worked with their current PCP to make changes in medications and therapy to help manage their particular conditions and individual needs. **Step 4 was completed.**

During this time, Linda spent countless hours on the phone questioning other caregivers, doctors and anyone who might have advice about what to do next. The scary and tough decisions continued to loom, and the most important was the financial aspects of how much all this new care was going to cost and could their resources pay it. Bernice and Gene came to us with a limited fixed income, no savings, and a substantial debt as well as a mortgage on their home in Washington; their home was in need of considerable repairs before the family could even think about putting it on the market. Thankfully, Linda's older sister lived next door to their parents in Washington, and she was the logical person to handle the issue of the house repairs and sale.

To keep Gene and Bernice occupied and mentally stimulated during the months they spent with us, we regularly took them to an Adult Day Care facility (Joe's Club in Melbourne, Florida). As I was retired from the military and home most of the day, I took over the care giving needs during the day while Linda was at work. Joe's Club turned out to be crucial, as they gave us invaluable information on geriatric doctors and different types of assistance that were available to us through different organizations. When Linda contacted the Department of Elder Affairs, she found that one of their Care organizations worked out of the same facility as Joe's Club, so that helped Linda decide which program to choose when that step was reached. They set up a home interview to explain what their agency could provide and to determine her parents' needs. The state's long term senior care program's goal is to keep their members either at home or in an Assisted Living Facility, when appropriate, rather than a much more expensive nursing home. We discussed financial issues and after we learned her parents met the criteria for financial aid for an ALF, we opted for their program. **Step 5 started. Note: It took 6 months and many applications before the State finally approved their application for assistance. Step 5 is the hardest step, requiring many applications and re-attempts, so DON'T GIVE UP!!**

With a clearer picture of what Gene and Bernice's income was and an idea of how much financial aid the managed care program would cover for an ALF, Linda and I started looking at the ALF listing that the program caseworker had provided us; we started to call and visit the ones that were in our price range and provided the different amenities and services that we were looking for in a facility. Different facilities provided different things. Some facilities were larger and provided many group activities such as daily exercises, games, entertainment and field trips. Some were smaller, more personable with a homier atmosphere, but did not provide as many activities/amenities as the larger facilities. Some had independent residents mixed with those that needed more assistance. Linda was very interested in facilities that also had a Memory Care Unit that would control the resident's movements so that if her parents should become a "wandering" risk, they would not be able to leave the facility without supervision. Linda and her parents settled on a list of about 6 facilities and visited them. Linda and I narrowed the list to two that they liked. One was small, homey and close to us, and the other one, although a little further distance from our home, was a larger facility with more activities, and also included a Memory Care Floor. After many visits and discussions on which facility would be better for them, Linda, her parents and I agreed on the larger facility; we negotiated a contract and arranged a move-in date. **Step 6 done**.

During this time Linda and her parents had met with an Elder law lawyer who specialized in elder care, who counseled them on the legal paperwork that Linda would need in the state of Florida to legally manage her parent's financial, medical and legal affairs. Of note: in Florida, a home or any equity in one is not considered as income or a financial asset, but check with your lawyer. We sat down and went over all of their financial information, to determine what their financial situation looked like, and what we would need to pay for their continuing care. **Step 3 and 7 initiated.**

Gene had also served in the Marines, so I contacted the VA to see if he would qualify for any medical or financial aid. I took him to the VA and initiated the application for financial and medical aid. Although it took a while, we found that he qualified for some medical care and, specifically, the VA audiology department was able to fit him with new hearing aids, as his hearing impairment correlated to his military work on a flight line in the mid-1950's, which left him with decreased hearing ability. Additionally, he was eventually qualified to receive a small monthly stipend, which helps with his various healthcare costs. **Step 8 initiated.**

As with any brain-centric disease, the Alzheimer's/dementia progresses, and Gene and Bernice are presenting more advanced stages at a rapidly increasing pace. Linda, I, their doctors and long-term case managers all continue to work with the agencies noted above to try to keep her parents happy, laughing and as healthy as they can be.

TERMS

The differences between Nursing Home Facilities and Assisted Living Facilities (ALFs) are important and should be kept in mind when looking at housing options.

Assisted Living Facility (ALF) is a senior living option for those who are in need of some assistance with daily living yet aim to live as independently as possible. There are many defined types of senior living, and assisted living would fall between an independent living community and a nursing home. A typical assisted living home might offer 24-hour monitoring of its residents and various support services such as medication management, bathing and dressing, while providing the resident with more freedom and privacy than a nursing home.

No federal standards for assisted living facilities currently exist, so each state defines an assisted living residence differently. There are some federal laws that exist that impact assisted living communities, but most oversight occurs at the state level. Many states are moving towards defining their assisted living facilities as such, but others use different terms such as residential care facilities or personal care homes. Two thirds of states use the term "assisted living." It is also important to note that some licensed assisted living facilities may care for other residents besides seniors, such as mentally challenged residents and those with special needs. These facilities provide supervision or assistance with Activities of Daily Living (ADLs); coordination of services by outside health care providers; and monitoring of resident activities to help to ensure their health, safety, and well-being. Assisted Living Facilities are for those persons where independent living is not appropriate but who do not need the 24-hour medical care provided by a nursing home facility.

A Nursing Home/Facility is for those who require constant (24 hours a day) nursing care and have significant deficiencies with activities of daily living. Nursing aides and skilled nurses are available 24 hours a day, and resident rooms are similar to those in a hospital setting.

Note: At the time we were looking for financial assistance with the placement of Gene and Bernice in an Assisted Living Facility, Florida Department of Children and Families ran a pilot program called the Nursing Home Diversion Program—this program was initiated to save the state money and to stretch the funding the state provided by providing care giving and healthcare services to qualified members that enabled them to stay in their own homes or an Assisted Living Facility. The goal of the Nursing Home Diversion Program was to provide quality home health care and community based services to delay or avoid long term placement in a nursing facility. This program was replaced in August of 2013 by the State Long Term Care Program which is now run by the state Medicare system.

The difference in these two types of living facilities is important to note because a Nursing home tends to be much more expensive than an ALF.

Activities of Daily Living (ADL) is a term used in healthcare to define daily self-care activities within an individual's place of residence, in outdoor environments, or both. Health professionals routinely refer to the ability or inability to perform ADLs as a measurement of the functional status of a person, particularly in regards to people with disabilities and the elderly. ADLs are defined as "daily activities that we normally perform on our own, such as feeding ourselves, bathing, dressing, grooming, walking, work, homemaking, and leisure." While basic categories of ADLs have been suggested, what specifically constitutes a particular ADL in a particular environment for a particular person will vary.

Instrumental Activities of Daily Living (IADLs) are complex skills needed to successfully live independently. These skills usually include: managing finances, shopping, handling transportation (Bus or car), meal preparation, managing medications and using the telephone. Assessing IADLs can help guide a diagnostic evaluation, as well as determine what kind of assistance an elderly person may need on a day-to-day basis. Managing IADLs is particularly important in caring for patients with Alzheimer's and other types of dementias.

Levels of Care (LOC) are usually determined by how many and which ADLs and IADLs a person can accomplish independently. This determination normally will dictate what kind of facility the patient needs and the cost of service to the patient. The more IADLs and ADLs the resident needs drives the amount of work the staff must accomplish, thus the more expensive the care. Levels of care help facilities simplify their pricing structure into "tiers"; when a resident requires more care, they go into the next "tier," and the cost of that tier rises. This policy avoids a constant reassessment of costs every time a resident's needs change. Levels of care are also convenient for the consumer: you know the pricing up front, and can avoid feeling "nickel-and-dimed" every time a change occurs in care needs. Although the components of each level of care vary from facility to facility, there are some basic guidelines. Many facilities use this tier system to determine a resident's required level of care. No cost-of-care fee applies if the resident is considered independent and doesn't require any help. This can also apply to residents who only need verbal instructions to complete the IADLs and ADLs. Prior to quoting a firm monthly fee, most facilities will require a "care assessment" on any new resident prior to their moving in (usually performed by their own nursing staff). This will determine at which tier level price they will start. Important Note: Although we found that the majority of ALFs we initially looked at for Gene and Bernice operate on a Levels of Care Tier pricing system, we have since had to move them to another facility. Bernice had become a "wandering" risk and we were not comfortable with the current facility's ability to keep her safely within the facility, in addition to the rising costs of their monthly rent due to the need of more assistance with their ADLs. We re-visited, quite by chance, a facility within the same distance to our home that does not operate on a Tier pricing system for ADLs, but a flat fee for either independent living or assisted living. This knowledge turned out to be invaluable, as within a year of placing Gene and Bernice in the Tier-based pricing facility the increasing costs of both their care in the Tier system coupled with the need to move them to a memory care unit were rapidly becoming unaffordable. Advice: **Do your homework! Look for both types of facilities, and understand that as your loved one's assistance level increases, so may the costs if they are in a tier system facility.** In some cases, your loved one may be able to afford those rising costs, and this may not be a financial factor for you. However, if your loved one is on a fixed income and qualifies for financial aid from the state to help pay for ALF costs, then this may be something that you need to factor into your ALF placement decision. When we were looking at ALFs for Gene and Bernice, if we had known and understood the difference in the financial pricing and costs of the facilities, we would have gone with a flat rate facility. Although the initial monthly rate may be higher than a Tier based price facility, if you are looking for a long-term care facility, you will be assured that the costs will not increase as the level of care needs increases. This becomes very important for loved ones with dementia-related diseases, as the further their disease progresses, the harder it is for them to accept changes to their daily routine. Having to re-locate Gene and Bernice after only a year at their former facility into a totally new and unfamiliar living environment (due to the rising financial costs of their care, but the current facility provided a more secure Memory Care program and safer environment) was a very painful and frustrating process for all of us.

Health Maintenance Organization (HMO) is a corporation that is financed by insurance premiums and has network physicians and professional staff who provide health care. You must designate and use a Primary Care Physician (PCP), and you must use their doctors.

Preferred Provider Organizations (PPO) are corporations that are financed by insurance premiums which contract with a network of "preferred" providers from which you can choose. You do not need to select a Primary Care Physician (PCP) as you do in HMOs, and you do not need referrals to see other providers in the network. Generally the premiums are higher for PPOs in the form of co-payments if you do not use their "preferred network providers."

Agency Contact Info:

Federal

Affordable Care Act (ACA)
www.healthcare.gov
1-800-318-2596

Social Security Administration
www.socialsecurity.gov
1-800-772-1213

Medicare
www.medicare.gov
1-800-633-4227

Veterans Administration (VA)
www.va.gov
1-800-827-1000

Federal Employee Health Benefits Program
(FEHB)
www.opm.gov/healthcare

1-877-372-3337, then press # to get to a
representative for questions

Department of Defense (TRICARE for Life)
www.tricare4u.com
1-866-773-0404, then say "help," then say
"beneficiary"

State of Florida

Florida Department of Elder Affairs (Serving
Health Insurance Needs of Elders-SHINE)
www.floridashine.org
1-800-963-5337

Aging and Disability Resource Center (ADRC)
through your state Senior Resource Alliance (SRA)
has information about available programs in your
area
www.seniorresourcealliance.org
1-800-963-5337

Florida Bar Lawyer Referral Service
www.flabar.org
1-800-342-8011 (charges a $25 fee for a
30 minute consultation)

Florida Law Help
www.floridalawhelp.org then type in "Elder Law"
Agency for Health Care Administration (AHCA)
ahca.myflorida.com
1-888-419-3456, then press 3

Florida list of ALFs and Nursing Homes
www.floridahealthfinder.gov

Florida Department of Children and Families
Automated Community Connection to Economic
Self Sufficiency (ACCESS)
www.myflfamilies.com/contact-us
1-866-762-2237, press #

Senior Resource Alliance (SRA)
www.SRAFlorida.org
Local 1-800-963-5337
National 1-866-757-0709

Ombudsman
ombudsman.myflorida.com/
1-888-831-0404

County

Brevard County Legal Aid
www.brevardcountylegalaid.org
321-631-2500